© **Copyright 2016 by Simeon Lindstrom- All rights reserved.**

In no way is it legal to reproduce, duplicate, or transmit any part of this document in either electronic means or in printed format. Recording of this publication is strictly prohibited and any storage of this document is not allowed unless with written permission from the publisher. All rights reserved.

Respective authors own all copyrights not held by the publisher.

When Life Gives You Lemons

- Squeeze 'em Dry

The Power of Surrender, Humor and Compassion When the Going Gets Tough

By: Simeon Lindstrom

Table of Contents

Introduction
Chapter 1 – The Best Laid Plans
- The "Thing"
- Planning That Disregards The Thing
- Planning That Respects The Thing

Chapter 2 – Embracing Change, the Root of Resilience
- Gritty Thinking
- Fragile Thought One: The World Is Hostile
- Fragile Thought Two: Life Is Elsewhere
- Fragile Thought Three: It's Hot To Be Perfect
- Fragile Thought Four: It's Wrong To Be Wrong
- Fragile Thought Five: There's Only One Way

Chapter 3 – How To Let It Go
- Letting Go Of The Past
- Letting Go Of The Present
- Letting Go Of The Future

Chapter 4: Inoculate Yourself With A Good Life Philosophy
- There is no Lemon: Ridding Yourself of 10 Common Cognitive Distortions
- Overgeneralization
- Emotional Reasoning
- Personalization
- Black & White Thinking
- Filtering
- Catastrophizing
- Prescriptive Thinking
- Mindreading
- Assuming Omniscience
- Sunk Cost Thinking

Chapter 5 – The Stoic's Recipe For Good Lemonade
- Step One: Acknowledge That Shit Happens
- Step Two: Be Reasonable, Leave The Drama Out Of It
- Step Three: Ask Yourself How Much Control You Truly Have In A Situation
- Step Four: Put Your Energy In The Right Place

Conclusion

Introduction

Ask a few people to tell you their quick life story and you may be surprised by a recurring pattern.

It's not obvious at first, but the person speaking invariably says something along these lines: "Well I was doing X, because I had planned for it for so long, and then I was going along, doing that, when Y happened, which was totally not what I wanted to happen. So I did Y for a bit and then had this idea to do Z, but after Q happened, stuff was just never the same again…"

You can substitute literally anything into that same story and have the life trajectories of most human beings. You were married and busy living your happily ever after when you met someone who changed the game completely. You studied for 5 years only to discover the field you were now qualified to work in no longer interested you. You expected a girl and got a boy. A windfall happened. You got in a car accident.

There are two things going on here: your plans, hopes, dreams, and beliefs about your life…

…and *life itself.*

Life, as they say, happens when you're busy making other plans.

We all have a narrative of ourselves that we hold dear, and when life "happens", we might feel a little slighted. How dare reality come and get in the way, just as we were busy trying to do our own thing? Nobody anticipates cancer, a surprise pregnancy, or being laid off of work. Nobody knows when they'll fall in love or when their uncle will die in a plane crash. But if you listen to the stories people tell, it's almost as though these random, unforeseen and unplanned for events were not distractions from life, but the main event.

"We never ever planned on having children, but it turned out to be exactly what we always wanted."

"I was very idealistic then. Ten years later, I don't believe any of that stuff anymore."

"I thought we would be together forever. I never even imagined that that could happen to *us*. Now I've moved on and found someone completely different."

This is a book about *change*. No matter who you are, there's a good chance that life has stepped into your self-made narrative and ruined everything, probably more than once. We like to shrug and write off events like this as "accidents". We like to focus instead on tinkering with our plans even more, or changing the narrative. Life knocks our tower of blocks down and we start right back up again, building another one. But is there another way to cope when life gives you lemons?

This book is also about *resilience to change*. Other self-help books out there may have mountains of valuable advice on how to construct your block tower beyond your wildest imagination. Personal development is usually focused on the tower: how can you build a better one? Why are you building one in the first place? How does your tower compare to other towers and is it normal? Is it a good tower?

These are all excellent topics. But again, they don't say anything about what to do when someone comes and knocks your tower down. You could spend years meditating, cultivating an inner calm and telling yourself a grand narrative about non-attachment and letting go of ego. But then someone breaks into your home and robs you at gunpoint and all at once, your narrative shatters. Your blocks are scattered onto the ground and you're left with an ugly truth: your narrative of life and life itself are simply not compatible.

This book is for you if you've ever felt like life has thrown you a curveball. It's for you if you've ever experienced an incredible loss and thought, "Oh god what now?" or felt like your best laid plans came to a screeching halt. In the chapters that follow, we'll be looking at a quality that is seriously underappreciated in the self-help universe: resilience. Here, we won't bother with any specific narrative, but rather take an honest look at what happens when a hurricane blows through your life and strips you of that narrative.

We'll look at how resilient people differ from people who are "fragile" and how changing your thoughts (i.e. your narrative) can change how you respond and adapt to change. We'll take a slightly different approach in these pages: there are no accidents, no unforeseen circumstances – only life itself. Change is not something to fear or work against, but something to embrace and move with. In other words, getting lemons is the default!

A few years ago, life dealt me an incredible blow. Something I had taken for granted for years was snatched from me, and almost overnight, everything I held dear was called into question. I felt small, fragile and helpless. I blamed myself, everyone around me and life itself. And like so many other people who get back up after life pounds them down, I was one day able to look back fondly at that time. Today, I am *grateful* for how awful that time of life was.

Whatever trauma, hiccup, mistake or accident you've experienced in your life, my hope is that this book can show you how to roll with it, with resilience, humor, patience and compassion. Change can be a blessing, or a curse. But it *will* happen. Over and over again. Whatever your path in life, this book is about devising a plan that will get you there, *realistically*.

Chapter 1: The Best Laid Plans

Some people have unimaginably huge spaces between what their day-to-day living actually entails and all the things they wish it did. They may look out over their entire lives and see only something that's getting in the way of what's most important: all the things still to come. These people are waiting for their lives to align with the picture they have of themselves. They're waiting for life to start, unaware of all the time that's bleeding away with every second. "One day" everything will fall into place and things will look how they're supposed to. Until then, their actual life is negligible, just some meaningless thing to pass on the way there.

Of course, there's nothing at all wrong with goals and dreams. Unless someone had the audacity to dream up an idea of life that didn't exist yet, mankind would not have made any of the fantastic advances it has over the millennia.

But far more people use dreams, plans and goals in a completely different way. While I can think of people who've had their lives do a 180 on them, I've also know people who seem to have things fall into their laps; the chaos of life seems to fall in their favor, they go with it, they seem "lucky".

"The Thing"

Before we continue, I want to introduce the concept of The Thing. I've kept it vague because, well, The Thing always *is* vague. You've already encountered the thing yourself, undoubtedly. The Thing is sneaky, unpredictable, a bit of a nuisance at best, a huge disaster at worst.

The Thing is the way the random, chaotic nature of the world expresses itself on us. Sometimes it has the face of failed entrepreneurial projects, health problems that spring up from nowhere, financial setbacks or losses. Sometimes it looks like a bit of luck, or some happy windfall that comes just in time, just as you were giving up hope.

The Thing is random and follows no rules. By its nature, you never know when or if it will appear, and when it does, its form is always changing. The Thing *is* change. It's those irritating few dollars missing from your budget somehow. It's the genetic mutation that means you develop cancer and your friend doesn't. It's the spanner in the works, the uneven cobble stone, the typo and the plot twist.

There is no preparing for or anticipating The Thing, but it's certain: it's always there. If you look back on your own life, you can probably see a few times when The Thing pitched up, shuffled around everything in your life and left again, leaving chaos in its wake. Some changes are small but others are literally life changing: you lose a spouse, a limb, or worse, a vision of yourself in the future.

Planning that disregards The Thing

There are two ways to make plans in life. The first is the one that's usually encouraged by every personal power seminar, self-improvement book or motivational quote. Here, you begin with the assumption that you are in control, and that if only you are assertive, confident and goal-oriented enough, you can whip your life into shape, into the thing you believe it ought to be.

You want to improve, and you do so with a plan. You devise a workout schedule, set yourself the goal of a new job in 6 months, or buy a bunch of books that promise to teach you how to play the piano. In a larger, more abstract sense, you operate with a strong sense of who you are meant to be, and how your life is meant to turn out: in your vision you are in control, and events unfold in just the way you want them to.

Sounds good! But we all know what happens when life refuses to play along: tragedy. Where life and your vision of life meet, there's friction. You injure your foot and your workout schedule flies out the window. After a few months you start to wonder why you even want to get another job at all. And you sit down for an hour of piano practice and a minute later your mother shows up at your house.

The Thing comes. There's nothing in your plan that tells you how to deal with it – in fact, your plan scarcely acknowledges the existence of The Thing at all. Now, you're on the back foot. You're in a reactive frame of mind, scrambling to make a new plan, probably a little mad that you have to let go of your schedule and do this other, inconvenient thing instead. Because you're kind of invested in a path once you're on it, you choose to ignore warning signs. Or, because you're so convinced of this one course of action over another, you fail to notice a third, even better option. When The Thing comes, you aren't expecting it, and so its presence is unwanted, and threatening.

Planning that respects The Thing

Then there is a second type of planning. Here you not only acknowledge that The Thing might appear at any time, but you actually build that fact into your plan. Instead of being a rigid, static idea of what reality must look like, your plan has a few squishy places; parts that can bend and fold and accommodate change.

You don't hold onto to this plan too tightly either, realizing that you might need a new one at any moment so you'd better not get overly attached. When The Thing comes, you are expecting it, and so it's not some scary, unmanageable development – it's more or less just business as usual. Because you weren't chained to your plan, and the plan you had was malleable, The Thing doesn't impact you as strongly.

In other words, you are resilient.

Chapter 2: Embracing Change – the Root of Resilience

How resilient are you?

Take a look at some of the following traits shared by people who make plans that go *with*, rather than against the changing nature of reality, i.e. The Thing. How many do you identify with?

"I very seldom lose my temper."

"I can apologize quickly if I see I've done something wrong."

"I would rather just try something out instead of wondering if it will work."

"I don't mind if people are a few minutes early or late."

"I always have a plan B …and a Plan C and D!"

"I'm happy to be spontaneous sometimes."

"I'm OK with not understanding everything."

"I don't bother myself too much with other people's expectations."

"I can think on my feet."

"I'm always open to suggestions and like to mix things up."

"Things don't have to be perfect for me to be happy."

"I can always laugh at myself."

Gritty thinking

Luckily, resilience is not some inborn characteristic – it's a skill that anyone can learn. And luckily, you'll get plenty of opportunities for practice, since The Thing is everywhere!

Learning to be resilient starts with the thing you have the most control over: your own thoughts. The way that you interpret and internalize events around you has a direct consequence for the plans you make, the actions you take and the priorities you establish. Your thoughts make up the narrative you tell yourself, and give you a blueprint for how to understand change, loss and adversity.

Below, we'll look at how you might be unwittingly entertaining thoughts that are actually making you more fragile, as well as ways to reprogram those thoughts into more flexible, realistic and adaptable ones. Some of the thoughts below may seem more familiar to you than others. Some you might even disagree with, but I encourage you to read on – the portrait of resilience painted here is not what we typically think of when we imagine a "strong" person.

Fragile Thought One: The World is Hostile

So let's start: what does it mean to be tough?

What do we really mean when we describe a person as gritty, or resilient, or robust? And how are they different from those who are weak, fragile and unable to adapt and change when the going gets tough?

If you're like most people, you think of grit as a kind of *lowered sensitivity*. Tough things are not easily affected by external factors, and can endure a lot before breaking. To be tough, we think, we must be able to stand strong and not budge with any adversity. We must be like steel or leather or something immovable.

While this is a good description of resilience when it comes to building materials, it's just no good when applied to human beings! The trouble with this model of resilience is that it makes resilience and sensitivity two different things, and you can't have too much of one without compromising on the other.

In other words, when you reduce your sensitivity, you do indeed protect yourself and make it less likely that change, adversity or unpredictability can hurt you. But in the process you also shut out all the good things that come with sensitivity: social connection, intimacy, creativity, the love and enjoyment of beauty or the thrill of sensing the world around us.

Building a wall and hoping it will do the trick to protect you is one way of being resilient, but it's not the smartest. When you focus on all the dangerous and unpleasant things in life that you have to defend against, you unwittingly tune into the worst that life has to offer, and simultaneously shut yourself off from the best. When you're in this reactive, "strong" state of mind, you scan for threats and limitations, rather than opportunities. You set up a self-fulfilling prophesy where you seek out the negative and say, "Look! See? I told you it was there!" when you find it.

Fragile Thoughts:

- It's a dog-eat-dog world. Do unto others before they do to you!

- The only way to deal with negativity is with more negativity.

- It's not OK to be vulnerable.

- Shit happens. If something can go wrong, it will.

- If I shield myself, I can't be hurt.

The above thoughts are actually surprisingly common, and that's why I've begun with this as the first of five "fragile" ways of thinking. Maybe you're wondering, how can this mindset be considered fragile? Isn't it the opposite?

The trouble with this way of thinking is that it isn't realistic. If you had some undetermined food allergy, you could treat it by vowing never to eat food again. Sure, it'll solve your problem, but only in the most superficial way. You need food, and just shutting down anything that looks like it might prove problematic isn't solving that problem, it's more or less *avoiding* it. This is a fragile way of thinking.

Many people experience loss or tragedy and decide that they will seal up their hearts and never open them up again. While this is understandable in the short term, the loss of the ability to connect with the world, yourself and other human beings is a very, very high cost to pay for that safety.

Lemony Alternative:

Resilient people, on the other hand, are not "tough" in the usual sense of the word. Instead of forfeiting their human vulnerability, they hold onto it, but they moderate the way they think about threat and risk. When you see the world as full of hostility, you close up and get to experience nothing at all. If, however, you see the world as filled with both good and bad, you courageously take on the risk of occasional pain – but when you experience joy as well, it's all the sweeter.

What is *really* courageous, is to abandon black and white thinking and have the bravery to be optimistic, and see the good in life, even though you have been hurt in the past. Here are some alternative thoughts:

- No matter how dire a situation is, there are always options and opportunities.

- The world is filled with good as well as bad – and I am capable of handling both!

- It's OK for me to suffer sometimes. It's OK for me to feel a whole range of emotions.

- Being vulnerable takes courage.

- I don't have to numb myself or lower my expectations of the world to be considered rational, grown-up or smart.

Fragile Thought Two: Life is Elsewhere

When life comes along and messes up your best laid plans, your very first reaction might be one of surprise. While it's true that some events really are out of the blue, most of the time, things develop somewhat predictably, and if only you paid enough attention, you might have seen how that situation evolved.

You *can't* see things evolving in front of your eyes if you're not looking, though. If your mind is firmly stuck in the past or the future, you may notice nothing in the present at all, and something might land at your feet "out of nowhere." It's as though life is most inconvenient when it forcefully reminds us of where everything *really* takes place: in the present.

You might have missed some signals, lost awareness or stopped paying attention and then *boom*, something happens and you feel blindsided. It's not necessarily that life is unpredictable, only that you weren't really paying enough attention to predict it!

For lack of a better term, you might be living your life *elsewhere*. In regrets from the past or in dreams or worries of the future, you live in anything but the reality of the now. This is a fragile state of mind to be in because it means you have diminished awareness, reduced control and less agency in the minute to minute events of your life. You make poor choices or fail to choose at all. And when things change up, you're not prepared. You feel cheated, rushed or disconnected from the things that are happening in your world.

Fragile Thoughts:

- I know just exactly how to live a good life and do everything I want – but I'll get started on Monday, just as soon as I finish XYZ...

- I wish I could go back and change what happened in the past. My regrets. My unfulfilled hopes. Such a pity. I dwell on these thoughts all the time.

- What if...?

- In the future stuff will be better.

- Because of the way things were in the past, my future is set and can never be changed.

All of these thoughts might have more or less validity to them, but they all miss one crucial point of focus: what can you *do*, right *now*? It's metaphysically impossible to take any action in the past or the future, so if this is where your brain spends most of its time, what you're doing is training yourself to be inactive.

Of course, human beings tell themselves stories, and to do that you need to to think of the past and the future. But resilient people choose the present moment as their primary habitat, and don't make a habit of dwelling in frames of mind that limit their scope of action.

Lemony Alternatives:

Pay attention. To be resilient, to have the best possible response when life gives you lemons, you need to be present.

- When I'm in the moment, I can think on my feet, be alert and tuned in to everything that's going on around me.

- My life is not going to happen some other time, in some other place – it's *already happening*, right now.

- I don't have infinite time on this earth.

- The past is over. The future hasn't happened yet. The only thing that is real is what is happening right now.

- The only way to "miss out" is to not be present in each and every moment.

Fragile Thought Three: It's Got to Be Perfect

I'm sure you've heard someone say that their greatest flaw is being too much of a perfectionist. While they might have meant it as a sort of humble-brag, the truth is that perfectionist thinking really *is* a problem.

When you cling to the idea that your life should be nothing less than ideal and that you won't rest until you've achieved perfection, it can feel very reassuring. In a chaotic world, you tell yourself you're OK: other people can be incomplete or slightly messy or change their minds mid-plan. But not *you*. You hold high standards and hope they'll protect you from failure, or insulate you against the unexpected.

But the irony is that perfectionism is actually quite a fragile state of mind. It's rooted in the fear of loss of control, and it's almost a little superstitious: "if I do this *just right* then everything will be OK…"

You might set your heart on growing a rare and delicate orchid, clearly a perfect flower if ever there was one. But the fact that your orchid can only grow in a very narrow, very specific set of conditions is actually a disadvantage. Holding onto the image of a perfect life or outcome feels like it should be motivating, but when you decide you'll only be satisfied with that narrow range of outcomes, what you're actually doing is signing up for a *wider* range of possible failures. When it grows, an orchid is beautiful. But there are many, many more ways for an orchid to *not* grow than for other flowers. The irony in being a perfectionist is that you actually end up courting more imperfection.

Fragile Thoughts:

- There is a final, finished, complete outcome that I am striving towards. I don't know what happens once I reach it, but presumably I'll stop and my mission will finally be over.

- All my happiness will come at the end, once I'm done. But not before. There's no happiness along the way, and I won't rest at all till my plan comes to fruition.

- If I am to succeed, I must be hard on myself.

- I would rather not do something unless I can be assured that I can do it perfectly.

- I'm not like other people – I have higher standards, more exacting tastes and for me, the stakes are just higher.

Lemon Alternative:

As we've already seen, shit happens. While it might *feel* good to have a rigid set of conditions for reality and for yourself, they usually don't do much to dampen the chaos or unpredictability of life anyway. Basing your happiness on a very specific and limited set of conditions puts you in a reactive, fragile state. And even if you *do* achieve that state for a while, there's no guaranteeing that it'll last forever. Even the perfect orchid has to die eventually. Chaos and imperfection are *inevitable*, and when they occur, the perfectionist is the least equipped to deal with it.

Lemony Alternative

Don't be perfect, be a work in progress.

When you are a perfectionist, you are intolerant to incompleteness. But the trouble is, the road to perfection is 100% made up of incomplete stages. That's basically all it is! The most sublime ballet performance is danced on the top of thousands of hours of ugly missteps, grubby dance shoes and sweat stained practice gear. This "imperfection" is not taking away from the glamor of the end result, it's *part of* the end result!

Try these lemony thoughts instead:

- Every single moment is full, complete and whole on its own.

- Life is not just lived to get to the end of it.

- If I am to succeed, I have to be OK with moving through the process of getting better and making mistakes.

- I don't have to do everything at once. I can be "on the way". Being "in process" is not a failure.

- If my standards prevent me from taking risks and doing hard work, then they are not perfect – they're restrictive and unrealistic.

Fragile Thought Four: It's Wrong to be Wrong

Let's build on the above fragile thought. Many perfectionists (and I used to call myself one, too!) are deathly afraid of failure. They don't want to be measured and found wanting. They don't want to try and make a mistake, and for others to see that mistake. They don't want second or third place. They don't want to get better by increments, but all at once and quickly, so they don't have to go through the awkward middle phase when they're still learning.

The core of this fragile thought is that it is undesirable to be anything other than all-knowing at all times.

Sounds extreme when you say it directly, but the idea is that all the struggles of learning are unacceptable, and if you try something, you ought to be good at it right away, even if you've never done it before.

Doesn't it seem silly?

Have you ever sat in a class or listened to someone explain something and thought, "damn, I'm stupider than I thought"? Have you had trouble with something new and unfamiliar, yet nodded your head when asked if you understood or pretended like something was easy just to save face?

Maybe this attitude comes from the days of teachers punishing students for not knowing the right answers. Who knows. The fact is, though, that no learning can happen without occasionally being wrong. Unless you can honestly admit what you don't know, how can you begin to know it? Unless you acknowledge something is a mistake, how can you do it better next time?

Fragile Thoughts:

- Being in error is embarrassing and something to be ashamed of.

- Looking like I don't know what I'm doing will undermine my credibility and people won't respect me.

- It's all or nothing – I don't want to try unless I can do it well.

- I'm the only one who finds doing new things difficult – and I have to conceal that fact!

- Doing something and then admitting you were wrong makes you unreliable.

These kind of thoughts are tricky because they focus on creating the *illusion* of control, all the while giving you less control. Think about it – if you're stubbornly refusing to admit mistakes, to do things imperfectly or to be a beginner in any way, you're robbing yourself of the opportunity to actually learn.

So, you end up saving face, but at what cost? Stubbornly avoiding the discomfort of learning means you stay longer with thoughts and actions that aren't working, and miss out on the better alternatives just around the corner, just hiding behind the admission of, "oops, that's not right, let me try again."

Lemony Alternatives:

- I don't have to know it all, and nobody is expecting that I do.

- I don't take myself too seriously – mistakes are kind of funny! I just laugh at myself and move on.

- There is no shame in incomplete knowledge, or having an only partially developed skill.

- Knowing something is better than *seeming* like you know it to others.

- If I want to be better at something, I have to be honest about all the ways I'm not actually there yet. I'm secure enough in myself that this doesn't bother me, though.

Fragile Thought Five: There's Only One Way

There is a saying that goes, "brittle things break before they bend."

There is a vicious cycle we can set up for ourselves when we try to deal with the innate unpredictability of the world. If we feel frightened and out of control, we may be tempted to clamp down and become more controlling – we make more and more plans, and those plans become more and more restrictive. It's as though we hope that with enough contingency planning and enough strictness, life can't ever get the chance to throw us a curve ball.

But when you try to constrain the natural unfolding of events around you, when you curtail spontaneity and try to force situations to be what they aren't, you end up with exactly the result you don't want. You realize how poorly real life fits into your vision of it, you realize how much work it is to maintain that vision. You paradoxically feel *less* in control than if you had held a little less tightly. You may respond to this by trying to exert even more control, and the cycle continues.

When you think about it, demanding that reality conform to your pre-made ideas of what it should look like is a little …arrogant. What's so good about your plan, anyway? Nobody can argue that making plans is a valuable human skill. But it's possible to take that planning mindset too far, and into territory where it doesn't really work.

Like the perfectionist above, making strict plans really only maximizes the possible outcomes that will make you unhappy. When you make a "plan", it might be a demand in disguise, a secret intolerance and a disappointment waiting to happen. You say, "I'll get married before 30" and feel like you're a forward thinking, take-charge person who's taking actions to get what they want. That might be the case, but is when you get married *entirely* under your control? Do you really want to sign up for the three necessary years of misery if you only end up married at 33?

The trouble with plans and goals is that they can have the effect of *constraining* you. You put blinkers on and stop yourself from seeing something better that's right under your nose, just because it doesn't fit in with the plan you've already thought through. You might fail to heed warning signs because you're already convinced your course is the right course. Not to mention that when you live your life to a tight schedule, you sap the joy and spontaneity out of it.

Fragile Thoughts:

- There is only ever one correct and true way to do something.

- Unless I'm constantly vigilant, everything in life is going to go to shit.

- If you have good principles, you should never go back on them, never change your mind and never entertain other possibilities.

- If I do it right, I can help people see the error of their ways and help them to do what I think they should be doing.

- My life plans and standards only work out if they're followed exactly.

Lemon Alternative:

You're probably noticing some overlap with this fragile thought and the ones that came before. When you strip away all the intimidating strictness and go-getter vibe from this kind of thinking, you get to the root it: fear of change. Fear of loss of control, or of the unknown. If you can plan and control everything, then there's nothing to fear anymore, right?

This is wishful thinking, because so much of life is 100% out of our control. Trying to make it otherwise doesn't make you diligent and tough, it just sets you up for failure. When your plans don't work out, you're left with nothing. Nothing but your strong feeling that life should have gone otherwise – not exactly a frame of mind that's conducive to creative, joyful solutions.

Lemony Alternatives:

- I cannot change certain random events in the world. But I am always in control of the frame of mind I hold, so I focus on that instead.

- With the right frame of mind, I can respond spontaneously and quickly to any change in the environment.

- I am more interested in what works, and what works right now, rather than some lofty ideal I have of how the situation *should* go.

- I am flexible, and I don't mind abandoning a course of action if it repeatedly looks like it's not working.

- I am calm and in control – of *myself*. It's not my business to control others.

Chapter 3: How to Let it Go

As we move on, I'd like to focus on an "anti-skill", something that isn't usually thought of as an aptitude we need to develop in ourselves. This skill is the skill of letting go.

Letting go of what? Well, everything.

Letting go of the past = forgiveness instead of resentment, despair and regrets

Letting go of the present = spontaneity, instead of being neurotic or controlling

Letting go of the future = trust, instead of stress or anxiety

Life, when it's doing its own thing, is remarkably ill-defined. It's loose, bursting with creativity and unpredictability. Life is transient and everything around us – including us – is temporary, and prone to being lost at any moment. Life flows and moves, never clinging to one particular form and never stagnating in one place for too long.

Trying to stand still, to stop up the flow or insulate yourself against change only guarantees that you'll be more unnerved by change when it eventually happens. To match life's pace, you need to *let go*.

Letting go of the past

Resentment and regret builds when we look back at what has already happened in life, and tell ourselves the story, "that *shouldn't* have been." The trouble is, of course, that what is done can never, ever be undone. When you do this, not only are you fighting with reality, but you're fighting with a version of reality that has long gone, and doesn't even exist anymore.

Holding onto things from the past is taking extra effort out of your life to keep alive a story that is already over. If we have experienced a trauma, our minds may be tempted to return back to the event over and over, perhaps in a bid to finally get some "closure", to understand what happened, to gain a measure of control over it.

But at the end of the day, the counter is reset and everything is shifted: what was real and present one moment is immediately past, immediately history. This flow is a natural state – the trees don't mourn the leaves they lost three winters ago. What is unnatural is to hold on. This takes more effort, because you are actively working against life's current. When you let go, you're letting go of your hold on something in the past, a thing that's likely taking you out of the present.

Forgiveness is one of the most straightforward things you can do ...but it is one of the hardest. There is no real secret to it. Closure is a myth. You never get to go back and change what someone did or said. All you do is decide, just like that, that you are not going to hold on anymore. Not because memories of the past don't hurt anymore, but in spite of the fact that they do.

Visualize ropes or cords that are binding you to a ship that is sinking. The ship will keep sinking, deeper and deeper into the past. And you will sink with it unless you have the courage to hack away at those cords and swim away. The problem is not the sinking ship – it will sink anyway. The problem is that you are tethered to it.

Letting go of the present

For the most part, it's far easier to get stuck with stressing about how things were or how they might still be. But if you're anything like me, then you find a way to distort even the *present* moment, too.

Rigidly holding onto plans for how the moment *must* unfold can be exhausting – and seldom even works. Loosely, people recognize this kind of mindset for what it is: stress.

But what exactly is stress anyway? In keeping with the theme of this book so far, I'd like to suggest that stress is often about fighting with reality. You're trying to do things that are sort of undoable. You're racing against the clock, or doing something that's just innately pointless or unpleasant, or you're out of control and badly want to be back in control again.

I won't try to suggest that every bit of stress you experience is just an illusion, but ...a lot of it is. Let go of it. If the reality is that you were meant to be in a meeting in 5 minutes, and you're 15 minutes away, well, there's no using fighting with reality. You will be late. Instead of using that extra 10 minutes to stress and be anxious, why not use it to accept the fact and do what you *can* do?

I'm convinced that so much of the stress we all experience is completely elective. You actively have to hold onto it. But what if you let go? The next time something in the present moment is stressing you out, ask yourself if your fighting against reality is really reasonable, and if there's a better way to spend your energy.

Letting go of the future

When you stress and worry about the future, what you do is construct a picture of that future first. You imagine what might happen, and then proceed to treat it as though it already has. If you're stressed about people's potential reactions to a presentation you have to give, you are telling yourself a story about what the future is.

Of course, nobody can say what will happen in the future. You can only act in the best way you know how, in the present, then wait and see. It simply isn't your business to decide ahead of time how events will unfold. You cannot predict other peoples' reactions to you, and you don't know what *their* vision of the future looks like. There are always going to be things you haven't considered, factors you don't even know about, complexity in cause and effect that defy the understanding of just one person in a web of many.

Having anxiety about what might be is unnatural – it is holding onto something that does not yet exist. Of course, you could lay out a million contingency plans, try to see what is in the present and make an educated guess about what might evolve in the future. But that's all it ever will be: a guess.

The terrible thing is that, unlike the future you're worried about, anxiety actually *is* real. The cortisol you flood your body with when you put images and stories in your head is actual a real chemical in your body; a chemical that can do real damage, right here in the present moment. When you act out of fear or the desire to control, you take unreal thoughts and convert them into real actions. You may bring about the very thing you're anxious about.

The future, whatever it is, will come when it comes. And when it does, you will respond in whatever way you respond. Whatever anxiety you wasted in anticipation does nothing to alter the speed at which the future comes, or what it is when it arrives. It only robs you of the only thing you have: the present moment.

Can you prepare reasonably? Can you find a way to act to the best of your abilities, given what you know? Sure. And once you've done that, let it go. There is no way to actually be in the future or the past – there is only being present and not being present. So you might as well be present.

Chapter 4: Inoculate Yourself with a Good Life Philosophy

There is no Lemon: Ridding Yourself of 10 Common Cognitive Distortions

So far, in getting to the heart of what to do when life doesn't go quite the way you want it to, we've been making a pretty big assumption. When I talk about The Thing and how disruptive it can be, I'm assuming that ...there is a Thing in the first place. I'm assuming that when you look at your life and say, "how am I going to solve this problem?" that there is even a problem there at all.

We've had a long look at fragile thoughts vs. more robust ones. We've seen that to start getting to grips with the shit life throws at you, you first need to change your mindset.

Gritty people don't necessarily endure any less adversity in their lives. In fact, they may experience more. But what's different is how they *interpret* the events around them. A fragile person thinks in ways that limit him and make life harder, whereas the more resilient person thinks in ways that keep opening up options and possibilities. They may never even "solve" their life problems in the way a more fragile person would consider satisfactory, but it hardly even matters.

I'd like to consider here the fact that for a more resilient person, the very definition of "adversity" is different. They have a different threshold for what counts as a problem for them. The same event that could send a more fragile person into a tailspin barely registers for them. Why is that?

Below, let's quickly look at some cognitive distortions – which is really just another name for a way to *create* a problem where there isn't even one.

Overgeneralization

You fail one course at college and so assume that this means you must fail every course at college. You get dumped once and conclude that the entire human race finds you repulsive. This is a neat way to take a small glitch and grow it into a full sized Lemon.

Try this instead: Be specific. Force yourself to be accurate when you speak "I messed up *today*, on this *one* task."

Emotional reasoning

You feel fat and ugly, so, therefore, you *are* fat and ugly. You feel offended by something someone said, so you believe this is proof that they deliberately hurt you, and that what they said was objectively offensive.

Try this instead: Feelings are just feelings. Remind yourself that feelings are always valid, but not necessarily true.

Personalization

Your company is doing really badly and downsizes – you get fired. Your problem is now one of unemployment, but you give yourself another problem: the sadness at being rejected by your superiors. You feel worthless.

Try this instead: Easier said than done, but try to remember that nothing other people do is ultimately because of you. Accept your responsibility in a situation, but be realistic: is everything that happens directly related to you somehow?

Black and white thinking

In an argument with your spouse, their criticism of you makes you hate them, when you loved them an hour before. You discover a new hobby or passion, and it suddenly becomes everything, and whatever you did before is nothing in comparison. In conflict, you see issues as right or wrong, and people as all-good or all-bad. No in between.

Try this instead: It takes strength to consider the grey, middle parts. Listen carefully for when you use "always" or "never" or other strong, absolute words like "perfect" or "hate". Life is complex. Try to hold both good feelings and bad feelings about the same idea – it is possible!

Filtering

You receive criticism for your work and suddenly feel that life has given you lemons. But you have focused on just a handful of criticisms while completely ignoring the hundreds of times you were praised. You have a filter on that basically only lets the problematic aspects of a situation get through!

Try this instead: It's a rare situation that doesn't have both good and bad elements. If you find yourself in a difficult situation, actively remember to look for the positives, too.

Catastrophizing

This is when you take something that is a small problem and turn it into a huge, massive problem – the biggest problem the world has ever seen, in fact. This also entails assuming the effects of a problem are going to be much worse than they are. Perhaps you botch a speech you are meant to give. That's a problem. But it doesn't mean that life as you know it is over, and that this is the worst thing that has ever happened to anyone ever.

Try this instead: Fast forward a year or five years in your life and ask if this problem is still going to be an issue then. More likely than not, the problem will be long forgotten and its effects, if there are any, are very minimal.

Prescriptive thinking

This is another common way to create a problem when there isn't one. When you have plenty of "should" and "have to" beliefs about life, everything that doesn't fit that cognition is automatically a problem. Rather than rethink the belief, you might be tempted to go into problem solving mode. You think, "My toddler should be talking by now" and so when they don't, you think something is wrong. You try to solve a problem that may not even be there. You think, "Men shouldn't cry" and so when they do, you now have a problem on your hands.

Try this instead: Be careful about making these kind of rules for yourself. Say instead, "It would be nice if..." and then work to make that thing happen. Look closely at your prescriptives – are they really true?

Mindreading

This is when you wrongly assume you have more information about other people's lives than you actually do. You might say, "everyone hates me" but really, you don't have some secret ability to know what they think and feel without them telling you.

Try this instead: Forget about what other people think and feel. That's their business. Look at what people do and say, and go from there. Stick to "*I feel...*" statements and make no assumptions about what others feel. If you're curious, reach out and communicate before you jump to conclusions.

Assuming omniscience

This is the bad habit of assuming that you know all the facts, can see things from all perspectives and have considered all possible causes and effects. Sometimes you can, but more often than not, individuals are only privy to more narrow understandings of complex situations. You might forget to ask yourself if there's something you're not thinking of. You might look at some complicated social interaction and jump to conclusions, forgetting that there are "two sides to the story".

Try this instead: Purposefully look for evidence that disproves the belief you have right now. Withhold making serious judgments until you know more. Abandon your own perspective for a while and try to see the situation from another perspective – you might be missing quite a lot of information!

Sunk cost thinking

This is a bit like having a problem, seeing that it's a problem, but failing to solve it because you've already had that problem for so long, so you might as well keep going. For example, it might feel easier to leave an abusive relationship that you've only been in for a year rather than one you've been in for 10 years, even though both might be very bad relationships. Likewise, you stick with a bad business plan because you spent so much money and time putting it together.

Try this instead: Remind yourself that however much time, effort or money you've put into something, it's *already gone*. Sticking with a bad plan because you're invested in it won't make it any less of a bad plan. In fact, all you're doing is making sure your problem lasts much longer than it needs to.

Chapter 5: The Stoic's Recipe for Good Lemonade

The ancient Roman stoics had some pretty amazing ideas about life. Their comprehensive philosophy is way more than this short chapter can do justice to, but I do want to look at one thing in particular: Marcus Aurelius' suggestions for how to solve general life problems.

I present to you here my own bastardized version. Some form of the following is probably the single most useful skill I have personally developed, and I can say that many others have found peace, clarity and a heightened sense of resilience when they think about problems in the following way.

Step One: Acknowledge that shit happens.

I've been coy and called it "lemons" or "The Thing" but yes, life throws some very nasty, very unfair and very horrid things our way at times. The Stoics were …well, stoic. They didn't see any virtue in going into denial or sulking or feeling entitled to a more comfortable life. Instead, they just started with the fact: life is hard. Adversity happens.

Step Two: Be reasonable. Leave the drama out of it.

There's a place for emotions. But for the Stoics, you needed a cool, calm head when making important decisions about your life. Virtue, for them, meant a degree of control over your "passions", and a reliance instead of ethics and rationality. You might feel mad as hell that life has thrown you the curveball it has. But so what? That doesn't change the facts. That doesn't mean you can't make efforts to behave in the most rational way possible.

Step Three: Ask yourself how much control you truly have in a situation.

Once your passions have cooled down, take a good gander at your problem. I like to divide every life problem into just three groups: the first is the category of things that I have absolutely zero control over. Think a freak accident, the fact that we all must die one day, or whether my crush likes me back. The second category is all those things that I have *some* control over. While I can't control having done something wrong in the past, for example, I can control whether I apologize right now and make amends. I can't control whether the other person accepts that apology, but I can control how I respond to them doing so.

Lastly, there are those things that I have complete control over. Now, there's no need to get too philosophical about any of this. Nothing is set in stone, but in my experience, one thing falls into this category again and again: your thoughts, behavior and attitudes. No matter what, you are always in control of those.

Step Four: Put your energy in the right place

Commit to only putting your energy into the second and third category of problems. Let's say my problem is that my wife has cheated on me. What category of problem is this? Well, I can't control the fact that she has. It's in the past for one thing, and for another thing, it's totally something only *she's* in control of.

Well, then what am I in control of? I have some control over whether she does it again, but that can never be 100%. Even if I forgive her and trust her to never do it again, it's still not entirely up to me. In a relationship, what happens is always the result of both parties, so this will always be the case. But my thoughts, attitudes and behaviors – these I *am* in complete control of. I can choose how to respond, what I say and what I do.

Now, because I'm mortal and don't have endless time on this earth, and because fighting against things I can't change is a waste of that time, I can choose to only focus on what I can realistically control. I stop worrying about what she will and won't do (not my business) or regretting what she has done (also, nothing I can do about it now) and instead focus on my thoughts. It doesn't really matter what I decide to do once I've rationally thought it through. It only matters that I've taken the situation and made the best of it. Of course I can feel a whole avalanche of emotions – but I don't allow these to get in the way of me making the best possible decision.

This technique sounds kind of simple, but try it the next time you encounter The Thing. It can be pretty hard to pull off when you're embroiled in some heavy emotions, feeling confused or pressed for time, believe me! But try it anyway, and see how much clearer you feel in spirit.

This little blueprint is a nifty way to rid yourself of all the "fragile thoughts" we discussed earlier, and gives you the dignity of controlling what you can ...and letting go of what you can't.

Conclusion

There is an African proverb that says: "When there is no enemy within, the enemies outside can never hurt you."

Resilience is not about being stronger than anyone else, or stronger than the adversity life throws at you. It's about being stronger than *yourself*, overcoming your own weakness and beating that "enemy within".

None of us has any control over the random and sometimes deeply unfair things that happen in life. But we have complete and absolute control over how we interpret these events, how we talk about them, how we feel about them and ultimately, what we choose to *do* about them in response.

I hope to have convinced you of a few things in this short guide:

1. Life hurts. Bad things happen. People die, relationships end and dreams are broken. This is not pessimistic or a mistake – it's just reality. The first step to being resilient is frankly acknowledging that the world isn't perfect, and life will never unfold in just the way you wish it did.

2. Once you can admit this, though, you can start to *embrace* change rather than avoid it or fear it. Change can be scary and destabilizing, or it can be an exciting opportunity to grow and evolve.

3. To be resilient, cultivate resilient thoughts. Look at your thinking and move away from those beliefs that immobilize you, leave you feeling powerless or unable to cope. Move towards thoughts and beliefs that focus on all the things you *can* do, right now, to adapt and thrive.

4. Let go of the past, and let go of anxiety for the future. Let go of unrealistic demands of the present. Lastly, let go of your own biases and distortions – all those thoughts that convince you that there is a problem to be solved when a subtle shift in focus would show you a completely different situation.

5. Develop your own, meaningful life philosophy to help you move forward with courage, humor and resilience. I've given a quick Stoic technique as an example, but go with a worldview that leaves you feeling energized and ready to flow *with* the changes of life, rather than against them.

When you change your focus and start to work deep at the level of your own thoughts and beliefs, a strange thing starts to happen: the random external world is just not that important anymore. You know who you are, you trust that you will adjust and adapt to life's challenges, and so you can take a step back.

You might even find yourself *relishing* the fact that your life doesn't always go to plan. After all, this is an opportunity to push yourself, to rise to the challenge and prove to your doubting mind that you can endure hardship, and you can flourish.

Adversity is then not something to avoid, or some unfortunate detour from real life, but life itself. Adversity can be understood not as something that cheapens life or makes it ugly, but which sweetens it and encourages the best from people. The next time the shit hits the fan, do something radical: be grateful and become immediately curious about all the amazing new things you are going to learn in trying to adapt to your new situation.

In the saying, "when life gives you lemons, make lemonade", there is no mention of what it was you were intending to make in the first place, or what you expected to be given instead of lemons.

But it doesn't matter! *Because lemonade is delicious.*